SELF CARE Is HEALTHCARE

IMMUNE SYSTEM
SELF
THERAPY

HOW YOUR
OWN BODY
CAN COMBAT
CANCER

ALEXIA PARKS
10TRAITS.org

Books by Alexia Parks

People Heaters: How to Keep Warm in Winter

An American GULAG: Secret P.O.W. Camps for Teens

10 Golden Rules That Guide Loving Families

10 Golden Rules That Guide Teacher-Mentors

How Changing Your Name Can Change Your Life

Rapid Evolution: Seven Words That Will Change Your Life Forever!

Parkinomics: 8 Great Ways to Thrive in the New Economy

Parkinomics: e-book

How Love Heals (First Paperback Edition)

Published by The Education Exchange
(SAN #253-0872)
973 5th Street, Boulder, CO 80302
303-443-3697 - http://alexiaparks.com

TABLE OF CONTENTS

About the Author

Alexia Parks is an inspirational speaker and author of nine books. Her book: **Parkinomics**, *8 Great Ways to Thrive in the New Economy*, was written while she was recovering from colorectal cancer and surgery. It became a business and motivational bestseller on Amazon.com.

Over the years Alexia Parks has written for the national desk of *The Washington Post*, been a NYC magazine publisher, and served as Director of Communications for 100 major daily newspapers at the Sunday Newspaper Network in New York City. As an entrepreneur, she established a national mentor-training program, called Focus on Success, for teachers and parents. In addition, she has been called "one of 50 people who matter most on the Internet," by *Newsweek Magazine*, for setting up the first electronic voting system on the Internet in 1995. In 2007, she became the first accredited BLOGGER at the United Nations Conference on Climate Change (UNFCCC) in Bali, Indonesia. She currently blogs for the *Huffington Post*, magazines, is Director of The Education Exchange, and is working on two new book projects.

Joel Rauch M.D. In 2010, Alexia Parks worked with Dr Longevity, Dr Joel Rauch (Rauchwerger) M.D. to produce a series of 10 easy to understand DVDS, CDs and books on *Whole Body Health*. Some of the information for this book has been drawn from the DVDs of Dr Rauch M.D. Website: http://DrLongevity.org

Introduction:

Four major themes run throughout this book.

#1. **<u>Boost Your Immune System</u>**. The most powerful anti-cancer mechanism is the one that Mother Nature gave us which operates around the clock. It is our precious *Immune Defense System Against Cancer.* Your Immune System is actually called that in medical textbooks. As you will learn here, it is the job of the **T-Cells** of your own Immune System to fight cancer.

#2. **<u>Reduce Stress</u>**. Stress, in all its forms and varieties, is the biggest threat to your Immune System. These include the stress of everyday life, emotional stress, and stress from environmental toxins. Even good stress has an impact. To help you understand how all-pervasive stress in your life is, I've included the Top 10 stressful life events listed in the Holmes Rahe Scale.

Life Event	Life Change Units
Death of a spouse	100

Divorce	73
Marital Separation	65
Imprisonment	63
Death of a close family member	63
Personal Injury or Illness	53
Marriage	50
Dismissal from work	47
Retirement	45
Change in health of family member	44

Chronic, <u>long-term stress</u> attacks the Immune System and T-Cells of your body through the body's own stress hormone **cortisone**. Whenever the hormone cortisone is evoked, *due to stress*, it targets the Immune System and breaks it down. Basically, long-term, chronic stress breaks down your Immune System and its cancer killing T-Cells. *Yes, medically, they're called Killer T-Cells.* Their mission is to kill cancer cells anywhere they occur in the body.

#3. **<u>Reduce Free Radicals</u>**. Both Chemotherapy and Radiation generate *massive* amounts of free radicals inside your body. A free radical molecule is like a bull running loose in a china shop. In excess, they can cause rapid aging of the body. **Indiscriminate, free radicals damage everything they hit, including the DNA of your cells.** Damaged DNA can mutate into a cancer cell. *In this book, you will learn how to use food, spices, supplements, and even visualization, to help "mop" up free radicals.*

#4. **<u>Use These Techniques for Prevention *and* Recovery</u>**. In short, the very reason you got sick is also the cure. So following the guidelines in this book will help both you, the cancer survivor, AND those who are supporting you on your healing journey. The methods are fun and easy to learn.

Be a cancer survivor! As you regain your health you will do more than survive. You will **thrive** with a renewed sense of well being.

The "TYPE C" Personality

In the 1950's, two California cardiologists, Dr Friedman and Dr. Rosenman, made a great discovery. They were the first to really show how the mind is connected to the body. They noticed that in hard-driving people, especially men, who basically never relaxed, their incidence of heart attacks was sky high, much higher than the general population. So they coined the term the Type A Personality, showing that on-going, mental stress is reflected in the body by disease, in this case, heart attack.

And then, the relaxed person, they called: The Type B Personality.

So the simplified mechanism would be that this hard-driving individual, with an executive type personality that never relaxes, is constantly evoking the stress hormone **adrenalin**. Adrenalin comes from the inside of the adrenal gland. And because all hormones in the body have target tissues, **the target of adrenalin is the heart!**

In the Type A person, the heart is under constant attack from this SHORT-TERM stress. The adrenalin response is also known as the *body's flight or fight response. This puts pressure on the heart and entire cardio-vascular system.* The blood rushes into the arms and legs for rapid response and the digestive system is shut down.

The new information in medicine is that there is another stress hormone from the **outside** of the adrenal gland. This hormone is called **CORTISONE. And the target tissue of cortisone is not the heart; it is the body's IMMUNE DEFENSE SYSTEM.**

Cortisone is evoked due to **LONG-TERM**, chronic stress. So the cortisone hormone is evoked in the Type C cancer personality, the *long-suffering* personality.

Dr Joel Rauch, who was interviewed for this book, wrote a book in 1977 titled: The Type C Personality. It was one of the first books to link stress and cancer. In part, this was because Dr Rauch was doing research in the lab at Baylor Medical College in Houston, TX where the role of

the Immune System's Thymus and T-cells was
discovered.

So let's quickly summarize here:

Our stress glands – called into action whenever we
experience stress - are called the adrenal glands. And
they have TWO separate parts: an inside, and an outside.
And they produce two separate stress hormones. The
hormone released from the inside of the adrenal gland is
due to SHORT TERM "fight or flight" stress. This hormone
is called adrenalin. In the Type A personality, the target
tissue of adrenalin is the heart and cardio vascular
system.

The other hormone, cortisone, is released from the
outside of the adrenal gland. It is evoked whenever there
is LONG-TERM stress. The target tissue of cortisone is the
Immune System.

**For this reason, it is critical that those with the Type
C personality change their LIFESTYLE to ensure that**

stress is minimized, *continuously*. As you reduce stress in your life, you BOOST your Immune System.

A strong Immune System is your best defense against cancer. As I mentioned earlier, in all medical textbooks, your Immune System is actually referred to as: "Immune Surveillance System Against Cancer."

So it doesn't matter how the cancer arises, or is caused. A strong Immune System can help check and kill cancer in the body through its thymus derived Killer T-Cells.

And, medically, that's actually their name: KILLER T-Cells.

The Story of Fiber

How many readers remember the TV talk show host Johnny Carson? He had a guest on his program many years ago, a psychiatrist named Dr. David Rubin. Dr Rubin had written the first popular book on sex titled *"All You Need to Know about Sex But Were Afraid to Ask."* It became a New York Times bestseller. It was the first to discuss sex in public, before a mass television audience.

After his appearance on the Johnny Carson show, Dr David Rubin disappeared for many years. And then all of a sudden, he came out with a second book. The book was on fiber in the diet. So everyone wondered why is a psychiatrist who wrote a popular book on sex, writing a book on fiber in the diet? A book on sex? Yes. But a book on fiber? It doesn't make sense.

Well, it seems that his own Dad, age 52, had cancer of the colon. And Dr Rubin wanted to help out his Dad. So he went to the medical literature and sure enough, the answer was right there in the medical literature, overlooked, collecting dust.

The medical article was authored by one of the most famous doctors of all time: Sir Dr Dennis Burkitt. Who was Dr Dennis Burkitt? Well, he was so famous that they named a lymphatic cancer after him, cancer of the lymph: Burkitt's lymphoma. This, plus, his other contributions earned him a Knighthood from the Queen of England.

Here is Burkitt's story. In his retirement, he was traipsing through East Africa, and made a seminal observation in Kenya. What he noticed was that because of old Colonial system of government set up by the British, modern day Kenya has two groups of people: the indigenous Kenyans and the descendents of the old time Colonials.

So Dr Burkitt's amazing discovery was that the rate of cancer in the two populations was like night and day: black and white. It was completely different. In the descendents of the British colonials, the incidence of cancer of the colon was sky high. In the native Kenyans, it was almost zero.

So Dr. Burkitt figured out that the difference was based on what they ate, or didn't eat. It was nutritional. It was because the British population, by force of culture, would eat a lot of refined, baked goods, such as tea and crumpets. By contrast, the indigenous population had huge amounts of *fiber* in their diet, from corn, and many different types of vegetables, including fibrous potatoes and yams *with their skin intact.*

So Dr. Burkitt wrote up his results. These results were published in the medical journals, however no one really saw them, or did anything about them, until Dr. David Rubin. And Dr. Rubin, of course, wanted to help out his Dad.

At the time, there was only one medical remedy for colon cancer: surgical removal of the colon.

However, Rubin was so impressed by what he learned from Dr Burkitt, that he wrote a book entitled: *The Save Your Life Diet.*

The focus of the book was on the use of **Wheat BRAN**, as *fiber* in the diet. Wheat bran is not a food. It has no calories. It is simply the outer shell of the wheat, and costs less than 50-cents for a month's supply. At 1 tablespoon a day, that's only pennies a day. And, its daily use could reduce the incidence of colon cancer from the human story! Tell that to your family and friends!

What's the connection between wheat bran and cancer of the colon? The short version is this:

We all have approximately two pounds of bacteria living in our lower GI system, our colon. Any excess bile from the liver, which is not needed to break down or emulsify fats, is sent to the colon on a daily basis. There, it is acted upon in the colon by those two pounds of bacteria. The bacteria look at it as food and will quickly turn the excess bile into a cancer producing compound called 3MC, or three methylcholanthrene.

Three methylcholanthrene is used in medical laboratories on a daily basis to produce cancers in mice so they can do research on cancer in a laboratory setting.
.

This daily production of 3MC, however, occurs in all people, every day, as a normal, daily, bacterial byproduct of bacteria living in the colon.

So, the basic logic here is to eliminate the cancer producing 3MC from the colon each day, using 1 tablespoon of wheat bran. This supports Mother Nature's need for regularity. **Wheat bran supports a daily bowel movement and clears the colon of the cancer producing 3MC each day.**

It's that simple! The daily addition of wheat bran to your diet does just that.

Here is what it does inside your body. The wheat bran is insoluble, which is good. This means that it does not

dissolve in water. It acts like a scouring brush to clean the mucosa, which is the lining of the colon and keep it free of 3MC.

PREVENTION Technique: If a person takes 1 tablespoon of wheat bran per day (at a cost of about 48-cents per month) they will be nice and regular and will constantly flush out the toxic cancer-producing compound 3MC from their colon.

1. Stay Connected To Community

Here are 10 EASY lifestyle changes that will support your healing journey:

Biochemically, it is known that when people get together, pain-killing endorphins are released. So is "feel good" serotonin. That is, *being with other people can boost both our spirits and release a flood of feel-good painkillers.*

The life-affirming benefits of community are many. When you join with others "in community" by attending social events, the theater, cultural events, or participating in a group discussion you diminish the health impacts of stress, anxiety, depression and loneliness. For cancer patients this information is especially important because, in treatment or recovery, you may be especially susceptible to loneliness or depression.

In fact, Harvard University professor David Eisenberg M.D., whose research on cancer survivors was made into a Bill Moyers documentary for PBS television. It showed that when cancer survivors were by themselves, they lapsed into depression. By contrast, when they spent time together with other cancer survivors, with family members, or out at public events, their spirits were greatly lifted.

A final note, remember that music, laughter, and funny movies also provide connection to the greater human community. These too will lift your spirits.

The Power of Music: In my own case, *my chemotherapy treatment required a visit to the hospital once a week, and a 24/7 infusion of chemo Monday-Friday. When I went to the hospital for my IV treatment, I took along an IPOD given to me by my granddaughter. It was loaded with her favorite music, which became mine too. I would dance my way in and out, and with headphones on, could hardly sit still in the chair. Time flew by.*

__The Power of Community__: I opted for two types of chemo. One delivered by IV once a week. The other was delivered by a 24/7 infusion Monday to Friday. I carried a soft plastic bottle in a fanny pack, and chemo was delivered through a tube into my arm five days a week. Friday afternoon at 5 PM, I would unhook the tube from my arm, take off my little fanny pack, and head for happy hour with friends. No one suspected that I was a cancer patient, or taking chemo. Monday, the tube would be reattached at the hospital. I had the weekend "off" to blend in with friends and community.

I INTEND TO DO THE FOLLOWING:

---

2. Use Aerobic Exercise
For a "Feel Good" Boost

Aerobic exercise has many mental benefits for cancer patients, including the relief of stress, anxiety and depression, because it releases "feel good" neurotransmitters: **serotonin, dopamine, and endorphins**.

What this means for you, as a cancer survivor, is that *by doing a minimum of 20-mimutes of aerobic exercise every other day, you can be put into the most POSITIVE state of mind. The euphoria from exercise will carry over into the rest of the day.*

In addition, endorphins are the PAIN RELIEVING neurotransmitters. **Endorphins** are the world's greatest natural painkillers.

Endorphins are **200 times** more powerful than morphine, as a painkiller. Endorphin release occurs whenever you reach a **continuous level of aerobic exercise for a minimum of 20-minutes**.

Serotonin and endorphin are the feel good natural chemicals for cancer survivors. You want both of these neurotransmitters working on your behalf!

And there is more to this story. You have Mother Nature's Whole Pharmacy inside your body. It's your own personal pharmacopeia, free-of-charge. Without a prescription, you can evoke the entire pharmacy that Mother Nature gave you.

As a final point here, in addition to releasing serotonin and endorphins, aerobic exercise will also stimulate the production of the neurotransmitter dopamine in your brain.

Dopamine is the #1 neurotransmitter for motivation and GOAL SETTING. A lot of cancer patients will lose their interest in life and throw in the towel. You are a survivor. You want this neurotransmitter working on your behalf. **So to get motivated, get aerobic!**

What *exactly* is aerobic exercise? Here is what it is not. It is NOT weight lifting, golf, tennis, or even football. It is not a stop and start activity.

How do you reach aerobic levels each day? The key word here is CONTINUOUS.

Aerobic exercise means the **continuous** use of oxygen for 20-minutes every day (or every other day, at a minimum). Aerobic exercise includes the following activities:

FAST walking, running, jogging, bicycling, and swimming

The key idea here is to chose one activity and to do it non-stop for 20-minutes. My favorite is fast walking because I can do it anywhere.

Aerobic walking is known as THE PERFECT EXERCISE.

How can you tell when you've reached aerobic levels through fast walking? The simple test is this: when you walk anywhere – even at a shopping mall – you will reach the point where you are barely able to talk to a friend while walking. That is, you will feel a bit breathless. You can still have a conversation, but it takes a bit of effort to talk.

I INTEND TO DO THE FOLLOWING:

3. Learn To Say "No" To Distractions

You are on a healing journey. Your job is simple: you need to break free of all those things that are not on your healing path.

Right now, what you need to know is that the more a person is focused on a goal the less they are going to be distracted by the demands of ordinary life.

For example, the following is a metaphor from sports, which applies 100% to you, the cancer survivor.

The great sports medicine psychologist Dr Jim Loehr began his career by studying two classes of athletes. The first were athletes of incredible talent and skill. The other, were athletes of lesser ability. He was perplexed by his observation that in many cases, the athletes of lesser ability beat the athletes of greater ability and talent.

He asked why. The answer was found on the tennis court. In a typical match, the athletes of greater ability were easily distracted. The crowds, the noise, the discursive thoughts going through their mind, the negativity of self-criticism all swelled up like a volcano inside of them.

By contrast, the more mediocre athletes used the 20 seconds of downtime in between points **to create their own ritual**. Some would never look at the crowd, or bounce the ball two or three times, or twirl their tennis racket. They would stay in the zone of inward focus. The ritual each chose was to guarantee the locking in of a focused state, without negativity, without distractions, without discursive thoughts.

Then, upon serving the ball, their mind would be totally clear and focused, and their natural talents would shine forth.

So how does this apply to you?
There will be many distractions in your life just like those of the superstar athletes. So what I would suggest is **to**

create your own life affirming rituals for everyday life.

These might include affirmations during meals to affirm that the food will nourish your body and restore you to perfect health. They might be rituals to keep you focused when you go out in public, or visit your doctor. The affirmations and rituals should always to be framed in the affirmative.

I INTEND TO DO THE FOLLOWING:

4. Visualize. See Yourself In Perfect Health

Did you know that you can actually program your mind for the goals that you want to achieve?

When programming your mind with a new goal, the secret is to always see the END result first, as already done, a fait accompli, finished! That is, see yourself in perfect health.

The reason for this is because of a phenomenon, called Eidetic Vision, which is defined as *intense mental imagery*. When in a relaxed, ALPHA state, your nervous system will automatically incorporate this visual programming into many cells of your body. You will learn how to get into an ALPHA state in Lifestyle Change #8

What does this mean for you, the cancer survivor?

This means that **whatever goal you set, needs to be visualized as complete.** Already accomplished! For example: you can visualize your Killer-T Cells doing their job; cleaning house, cleaning up all of the residual cancer cells. So, for example, if you have radiation or chemotherapy treatment, which can kill up to 95% of the cancer cells, you can then use an intense visualization to mop up the remaining 5%.

As a reminder: up to 95% of cancer cells can be killed with chemotherapy and radiation. To reach 100% kill rate, a person would have to be given such a strong dose that it might also kill that person.

In a sense, it is like calling an exterminator to your house to rid it of bugs. The exterminator may tell you: "I can hit these three spots and kill most of the bugs. If you want 100% of the bugs killed, I will have to use such a high dose of toxic chemicals that it would severely affect the people living in the home." Of course, you would say OK to the method that would kill the 95% of the bugs.

Harsh radiation, like X-rays, is known to kill cancer cells. Certain chemicals – called radiomimetic drugs – mimic radiation, and also kill cancer cells. So what is done is give chemotherapy and/or radiation to kill 95% of the cancer cells. Then the goal would be to apply alternative therapies. You can use Mother Nature's ability to do the final reconnaissance and mop up the remaining 5%.

The basic technique is to do **intense visualization while in a relaxed ALPHA state.** This will decrease your cortisone levels, and help activate your Immune System, especially your Killer T-cells.

Your goal is to visualize your own Killer T-Cells killing the remaining 5% of cancer cells. That is their job. They are doing what they were designed to do. **Conscious visualization while in the ALPHA state works like magic because visualization at this level helps activate Killer T-cells.**

The visualization that I used during radiation therapy was to imagine that the cancer cells were being spiraled out of my body and sent up into the sun, where they would instantly burn up.

For many cancer survivors, their mind is always thinking cancer, cancer, cancer. Instead, they need to go back home to Mother Nature. They need to remind themselves: **"I am in perfect health."**

Mother Nature isn't logical. Love isn't logical. She will support whatever you imagine... in a relaxed state.
Image this: "Mother Nature loves me. Mother Nature supports me, every second. Mother Nature has made me perfect in every way."

This could even be taken on a spiritual, transcendental level. On this level, the Cybernetic mind, the goal-setting mind, kicks in. Suggestions: verbal and visual, sink in.

The more intense the Eidetic Image, the more it will sink in. The more confidence you have in the process, the more it will sink in. The more senses you bring to the imaging, the more it will sink in.

Biochemically, what seems to happen is this: when you get down to the alpha state, your cortisone level decreases. When you are in the alpha state, which is about 10 cycles per second, you evoke the natural healing rhythms of your PARA-sympathetic nervous system.

The Para-sympathetic nervous system is the receptive state, the YIN state, the state where the seeds of positive images and suggestion will take hold in your subconscious mind. They will take hold, take root, and grow.

If your body is in resistance, nothing will take. If your body opens up, relaxes and is receptive, the images will take hold and grow.

Another term is FAITH. Or, Confidence. Go with faith and confidence.

Even if you don't believe it, do it anyway!

I INGTEND TO DO THE FOLLOWING:

---

5. Make Time Each Day For Core Exercise & Stretching

Most people who have cancer are adults and senior citizens. So it's important for them to have a healthy mind and a healthy body. The fundamental connection of body, mind and spirit, is something that everyone involved in holistic medicine agrees upon.

So if we focus in on the body of cancer patients, especially the body of an older patient, it is very important to develop flexibility, balance, and core strength through stretching because this type of non-aerobic exercise gives the cancer patient a fundamental sense of well being.

Flexibility is especially important, because cancer patients may have a tendency to fall, lose their balance, or get disoriented during or after treatment. So any type of yoga, Pilates, core and flexibility exercise is important for cancer survivors. If you like, you can use common household props as a stretching aid, exercise balls, and even simple rubber tubing.

For example, if there is a chair, use it as an aid for stretching. If you stand against a wall, extend each arm upward and stretch your body against the wall. In other words, you can use common ordinary every day things as an aid for stretching and flexibility.

When I take my dogs out for a daily walk, I even use the back bumper of my car – with the back hatch door open – for a stretching prop. With the dogs patiently watching me, I do a few minutes of stretching before driving home.

All of these exercises automatically reduce stress in your body, which then reduces your cortisone levels. Reducing cortisone levels helps strengthen your Immune System.

Remember: when you use stretching exercises to gain flexibility and take stress away, you automatically help the Immune System recover.

What these stress free activities have in common is that they help TURN OFF THE MIND. They help shut down the stressful, negative thinking of the mind. They shut down depression. In the process, you will find yourself so engaged in the activity that you have chosen, that it's almost impossible to conjure up a negative thought.

In addition, and again on the positive side, **you will be releasing the powerhouse of endorphins, serotonin and dopamine**. Working together, these three life-affirming hormones create a very powerful ally for your Immune System.

I INTEND TO DO THE FOLLOWING:

6. Boost Your Confidence With A Reward System

Biofeedback technology is perfect for use in cancer therapy. *Biofeedback technology is simply a mechanical device that accurately tracks our progress in reducing stress.* Because it boosts our confidence level every step of the way, it is a technology that people love.

The basic concept is that Mother Nature gave us many feedback systems in the body. For example, you're hungry or thirsty, so you'll eat or drink. Once that thirst or hunger is satisfied, that mechanism will shut off.

When you are suffering from long-term stress, your body continuously releases the stress hormone, CORTISONE. And, the target of cortisone is the T-Cells of the Thymus, that is, your Immune System. When you experience long-term stress, the cortisone will continuously break down your Immune System and its life affirming T-Cells.

So any technique you choose, whether biofeedback, meditation, or relaxation, to reduce stress will preserve your Immune System.

Why? The heart of the biofeedback machine is this: whenever we relax or meditate, the machine will give us a feedback to tell us if we are doing the right thing. This constant feedback assures us that we are gaining the benefits we seek, through relaxation.

There are three major types of biofeedback.

If the biofeedback machine is attached to the scalp with a headband it is called Electroencephalograph (EEG) and will monitor your brainwaves. As you relax, your brainwaves slow down.

The second type biofeedback is the Electrocardiogram (EKG). You are rewarded when you slow down your heart.

The third type of biofeedback is called EMG. EMG refers to the muscles. This biofeedback technology is attached to your muscles.

So if you are measuring either your brain, your heart or muscles, the machine will give you a feedback response when you slow down your brainwaves, your heart rate, or when you relax your muscles.

The machine will give you feedback either as a sound or a sight to let you know that your body is relaxing. The more you relax and slow down your brainwaves to alpha state, slow down your heartbeat, or relax your muscles, you get a little "visual cookie," a little sound bite, or other sensory feedback as a reward.

Remember: it essential for you, the cancer survivor, to use biofeedback technology to learn how to consciously break free of chronic stress as part of your recovery therapy.

Can you substitute meditation techniques? Yes, but not at first. With meditation, one never has actual proof that they're doing it right.

By contrast, **the biofeedback technology's reward system is immediate proof from your body that you are doing it right.** It is proof positive that you are actually learning stress relief techniques. It's a confirmation that you're getting it right. You want to be right!

So, go for the confirmation and go with the machine. It will give you positive feedback when you're doing the right thing. As a confidence building factor, you want absolute proof that you are on the right track.

Practice makes perfect. Over and over it shows that you are reducing stress. And just like magic, your Immune System will respond. *Specifically **your Killer T-Cells**, whose job it is to kill cancer cells, will get back to work.*

Here's another benefit. When you use EEG biofeedback for your brain and learn how to quickly get into the alpha state, then you can also USE that alpha state for intense visualization.

Remember: Visualization works BEST when your brain is in an alpha state. When the brain is open and receptive, a suggestion, either LEFT brain verbal, or RIGHT brain visual, will sink in the best.

This is why it is critical for you, the cancer survivor, to have the certainty of the biofeedback technology. It's a life insurance policy.

Meditation is basically biofeedback without the machine, *without clear confirmation* that you got into an alpha state. However, you can use the confirmation of the alpha state through biofeedback to make a lot of progress. So start with the machine, and then, if you like, make a transition to meditation techniques.

Another way to block negative thinking and get into a meditative state is through repetitive motion or sound.

Repetition of any thought, sound, or motion will bring you into an alpha or trance state over time. Examples might include a mantra repeated over and over, or the repetition of a motion such as jogging or swimming. The very boredom of the repeated mantra, of the beat of your feet on the ground, or the swimming stroke, will drive you into an alpha state. In that state, you lose track of time.

When you lose track of time, you're in the alpha state. You don't notice the stress or pain of long distance exercises whether engaged in a marathon, or long distance swimming.

So if you're a cancer patient and don't have access to a biofeedback machine, take a long walk and pay attention to your feet, because the repetitive sound of your feet on the ground – shhhh, shhhh shhhh – will drive your mind into an alpha state.

Remember: meditation itself is stress release, as I mentioned, but don't stop there. Use that alpha state for conscious visualizations and suggestions about feeling GREAT, living cancer free, and being in PERFECT health, because that's when positive suggestions will sink in the best.

Use Operant Conditioning to control stress

For the cancer survivor, the key learning method is Operant Conditioning. For example, a child is good, so they get a reward. They get a reward for doing the right thing. A dog follows a command and gets a reward. In each case, the behavior is shaped by constantly rewarding the good behavior.

Operant Conditioning, using biofeedback technology, is used to shape inside behavior, those things that happen "automatically" on the inside of your body.

For the cancer survivor, the Operant Conditioning should be directed INWARD, toward the visceral organs, and the autonomic nervous system. Why? Stress happens real fast. Before you even know it, it hits the visceral organs and the autonomic nervous system inside the body. Your goal is to learn how to stay calm and focused at times of high stress. Your body will gain the benefits.

NOTES TO MYSELF. I INTEND TO DO THE FOLLOWING:

7. Eat Foods That Say "*I Love You*" To Your Body

Let's begin with digestive basics for the cancer survivor.

After any chemotherapy, radiation, or antibiotics, it is essential for you take one capsule of probiotic acidophilus daily for two weeks, to reestablish the friendly bacteria in your GI (gastro-intestinal) track. *(I use Nature's Bounty Probiotic Acidophilus which does not have to be refrigerated.)* After two weeks, you can return to two capsules a week.

And there's more digestive news you should know. At age 60, on average, 60% of your digestive juices are gone. Whatever your age, you need to pay close attention to what you eat, and in what order. At each meal, it's important to start first with protein. In addition, at any age, you will need to learn how to avoid diluting the digestive juices in your stomach with water, coffee, tea, soup, wine or beer when eating a meal. If a meal or snack includes *too much sugar, salt, or unripe fruit, it may bring on a sudden, unwelcome bout of diarrhea as the body does a quick cleanse.*

As a rule of thumb, **all liquids should be enjoyed up to 30-minutes before a meal, or at least 30-minutes after.** If necessary you can take digestive aids such as: Hydrochloric acid (HCL) to digest protein in your stomach; ox bile to digest fats and oils in your liver; and pancreatic enzymes to help digest carbohydrates. You can buy these separately, or combined as one digestive pill. These are all non-prescription.

For cancer survivors who have lost their appetite and need emergency anabolic nutrition, the strategy would be to take in as many calories, protein, and nutrients as possible, in a predigested form. The two major products that satisfy this requirement are: Isocal, and Sustical. They are intentionally made for cancer patients because they are loaded with nutrition. They are predigested so your body can quickly and easily absorb what it needs.

In general, for protein, you can enjoy any type of beef, chicken, fish, milk or eggs. You can also enjoy any type of nuts. Even Nutritional Yeast can be used to boost your protein intake.

For carbohydrates, chose any type of vegetable or fruit that you like, and **small to moderate** amounts of whole grains like whole grain rice or whole grain wheat, or whole grain oats.

If possible, your diet should also include two known, and powerful antioxidant spices such as turmeric (also found in curry) and ginger.

What is absent from this diet is large amounts of highly refined carbohydrates such as overcooked pasta, breads, cakes, cookies, donuts, pies, and sodas sweetened with fructose corn syrup.

The lifestyle diet I use is particularly strong in focusing on foods that are known as antioxidants. Antioxidants are known scavengers of free radicals. Quickly digested in blended form, these antioxidants go to work inside your body to mop up the free radicals created by radiation and chemotherapy.

What are free radicals? Free radicals are molecules in your body that cause extensive damage to all cells of the body. They come from every day living. For cancer patients, they come additionally from chemo and radiation therapy.

You can reduce the amount of free radicals by using anti-oxidants found in fruits and vegetables, red wine, spices such as tumeric, ginger, and cinnamon, and super vitamins such as alpha lipoic acid, and Vitamin C with bioflavinoids.

In the lifestyle diet I use, the centerpiece of my lunch and dinner always includes a **nutrient dense, antioxidant green drink**. Antioxidant also means "anti-aging."

Here is the recipe that I use. It is great tasting, costs only pennies a day and takes only a few minutes to prepare.

In addition to reducing the free radicals, it is a nutrient dense, easy to digest drink that will nourish your body in many ways.

Alexia's Super Antioxidant Green Drink

Place in a blender.

1 clove of garlic
1/4 - 1/2 **dark red** bell pepper
3 **sweet** pickle slices (plus a splash of sweet pickle juice)
Salt and pepper to taste. (Add turmeric, if desired)
Water (1-2 tablespoons)
BLEND (10-15 seconds).

ADD & BLEND: A handful (or two) of Baby Spinach.
POUR into wine or decorative glasses and serve.

OPTIONAL (My blender is a VItaMix. *I also add the following four ingredients into my green drink, stir in with a spoon, and enjoy each day at lunch and dinner*):

2 TBSP Oat Bran (or Psyllium,*for stool formation)
1 TBSP Wheat Bran (if constipated.)
1 TBSP Lecithin (supports the brain and cardio system)
I TBSP Nutritional Yeast (rich with full spectrum B-vitamins and protein).

*NOTE: If you use Psyllium powder, you must drink the green drink immediately. Oat and wheat bran allow you to sip it slowly, over a mealtime.

This twice daily green drink also includes plenty of **Vitamin A**. Vitamin A is known to reduce skin cancers, *both* on the outside of your skin and inside. When your skin turns inward, it is called: mucosal lining.

Why do I blend my salad into a drink? *The human digestive system can only extract a small amount of nutrients, 5% to 15%, from a raw vegetable salad.* The rest is processed as fiber. As a senior, with reduced digestive enzymes, I now get 100% of the benefit by blending my greens into a drink.

The POWER of protein.

Most important, for you, the cancer survivor is to build up and strengthen your body as fast as possible. The term used here is anabolic, meaning, to build up the body. *And what builds up the body the fastest is protein.*

The word protein means "of first importance", because protein makes up your muscles, your bones (95% of your bones are made up of protein; 5% calcium), your enzymes, your antibodies, your cartilage, tendons and ligaments. *Your whole body and your whole body chemistry are dependent upon protein.*

Since many cancer patients tend to lose their appetite after chemo and radiation, the idea is to take in the very best protein, the highest quality protein that is extremely easy to digest.

One protein that satisfies these criteria perfectly is the common cage-free EGG. The egg holds the GOLD standard for protein. The protein is in the egg WHITE.

The egg white, called albumin, has a protein rating of 100%. All other proteins like beef (about 82%), or chicken and fish (about 75%) are rated relative to eggs. Nutritional yeast, often used by vegans, offers 7 grams of protein in each 2 tablespoons.

In addition, the yolk of the egg is the only major *food source* for the essential Vitamin D-3. Vitamin D-3 is known as the "Sunshine Vitamin." Vitamin D-3 has over

20 functions including helping prevent cancer, especially cancer of the prostate gland. I take 2,000 I.U. of Vitamin D-3 in the winter months.

If you enjoy a 2-3 minute soft boiled egg that would be the BEST. I cook my 3 eggs a day for 3-minutes, then pour them into a bowl and stir. To me, it tastes like Chinese egg drop soup. I season this "egg drop" soup with salt and pepper, and then drink it directly from the bowl. Eggs can also be blended into a fruit smoothie. Avoid overcooked eggs, such as hard-boiled eggs. Overcooking denatures the protein.

The POWER of fish oil.

Omega 3 (DHA & EPA) fish oil is also referred to as Vitamin F. Whenever something is designated as a Vitamin, it means it is an essential nutrient for the body; lack of which – by definition – causes a major disease. So for cancer patients please make a special note to include a daily dose of Vitamin F.

Any fish or fish oil with a Nordic, or Icelandic, name in the label is a good choice. *To reduce the risk of toxins, I always choose Omega-3 fish oils from the clean, cold waters of northern countries like Norway or Iceland.*

Many nights, I enjoy (or share) a tin of King Oscar sardines from Norway, which has 2.5 grams of Omega-3. To boost daily doses of Omega-3 to 2 grams or higher, I include 1-tablespoon of Carlson Fish Oil, or Barlean's purified Omega Swirl, or Omega 3 fish oil capsules at mealtimes.

OMEGA-3 DHA & EPA (2 grams daily) is a daily insurance policy. It reduces inflammation in your body; feeds your brain; AND boosts your "feel good" serotonin levels.

Use these life-affirming guidelines for food to boost your mood, your energy, and most important, your Immune System.

I INTEND TO DO THE FOLLOWING:

8. Find Deep Relaxation With Massage & Sleep

At the University of Miami Medical School, the Director of the Institute of Massage, Tiffany Fields, has been studying the therapeutic effect of massage on cancer patients. Her work shows that in ALL cases, touch has hundreds of different benefits. Benefits include releasing endorphins and serotonin. In our society, however, still to this day, many people have the taboo against touching someone else. But touch is as basic as food and air to human beings.

On a practical level you can even do self-massage. And if you like, for less than $50, you could simply buy a massage machine. The kind I use is called HoMedics. The company has a whole line of very inexpensive massage machines. Because, on one level, *when you get a massage from someone else, or you do self-massage, what happens is you reduce the cortisone levels.* Touch reduces the stress hormone levels, especially the hormone cortisone.

Remember: the target of the stress hormone, cortisone, is the Thymus and its Killer T-cells. And the biggest KILLER of your T-cells is the stress hormone CORTISONE.

The T-cells that originate in the thymus are the body's police force. Their job is to keep cancer cells under control. The POLICE stations where T-cells hang out are the lymph nodes. T-cells are on constant police surveillance. They go round and round in the lymphatic vessels through the whole body, looking for cancer cells to control. Whenever there is a breakout of cancer cells, the nearest, local police station sends out the T-cell cops. It's that simple.

Your Immune System constantly checks for cancer regardless of how it is formed, whether it comes from chronic physical or emotional stress, constant fear or negative thinking, the sun's ultraviolet rays, or even environmental toxins such as pesticides. And what kills cancer cells? The T-cells that originate in your thymus.

You need T-cells to kill cancer cells. So, for cancer survivors, the name of the game is to build up your Immune System by not evoking the cortisone response.

You can do this when you:

1. **Reduce your cortisone level** by reducing stress in all its forms and varieties, including negative thinking. Find and hold positive images in your mind.

2. **Take Vitamin C with bioflavinoids** to build up your Immune System.

3. **Take the mineral Zinc.** Zinc is basic for the health of the skin, which is the body's first line of defense. A good skin without any breaks or lesions is important to prevent germs from getting into the body. Zinc also facilitates wound healing, and prevents stretch marks.

4. Enjoy a daily SELF-massage. One big way to reduce stress is with daily massage. Even a one-minute massage helps.

Massage is a sleeper, in the sense that it is one of those things that is basically free. You can do self-massage 10 times a day if you like, using any kind of oil. You don't need expensive oils. Any oil will do.

What kind of oils? These might include the cheapest vegetable oils that stay liquid at room temperature. Remember, you are not using this oil for consumption. It is for external use only. You can then wipe it off with a towel or take a shower. At some stores, specialty massage oil might be as high as $10 for 1 to 2 ounces. The choice is up to you.

Why should you use oil, as opposed to an oil free massage? Oil helps reduce friction, and thus enables a deeper level of massage.

5. Get a good night's sleep. For cancer patients, getting a good night's sleep is especially important because of the secretion during sleep of the master hormone called HGH (Human Growth Hormone). **HGH rebuilds all of the protein structures of the body,** *not only your muscles and bones, but also the antibodies of your Immune System.*

As you noticed, one of the great mega themes of this book has been keeping the Immune System as close to 100% as possible. And, the building blocks of the Immune System are protein, which is laid down under the influence of HGH.

Mother Nature produces HGH mainly during sleep, in just the amounts you need. The greatest pulse of HGH occurs just before 7 hours and 15 minutes of sleep.

I INTEND TO DO THE FOLLOWING:

9. HELPFUL SUPPLEMENTS

Cancer survivors need to know this: There are known foods and supplements that have an anti-cancer effect. Some of them are quite common.

1. Vitamin C with bioflavonoids. Vitamin C is known as ascorbic acid. Vitamin C always needs its helpers, which are called co-factors. And these co-factors are the bioflavonoids. For example, in the white of an orange, right under the skin, there are over 200 bioflavonoids. In addition, the most prevalent protein of the body is called COLLAGEN and only Vitamin C can make collagen. You need collegen!

Collagen forms the tight matrix of the body. It's the "white stuff" that makes up your body, not your muscles. And this tight matrix of collagen is one of the body's

MAJOR defenses against the spreading of cancer, called metastasis.

If you like, you can buy a Vitamin C (500 mg) *with* bioflavonoids, and then buy, in bulk, a powdered Vitamin C to boost your intake to 1.5 – 2.5 grams a day.

2. Zinc is needed by your Killer T-cells for maximum skin protection against cancer.

3. Vitamin E plus selenium. Most topsoil is deficient in selenium. It is know to work synergistically, that is, beneficially, with Vitamin E. It helps Vitamin E reach its maximum benefit for the body. So whenever you buy Vitamin E, make sure it includes Selenium.

4. Nutritional Yeast. The old yeast of the past was called Brewer's Yeast. When it is "tweaked" for human benefit, it is called Nutritional Yeast. Nutritional Yeast is the latest, beneficial generation of Brewer's Yeast. Nutritional Yeast is **50% complete protein**. If you are a vegetarian or vegan, you can get a high quality protein through

Nutritional Yeast. *It also has all of the B-vitamins including the most expensive one, B-12, in high, almost MEGA doses.* In addition, it has 17 different minerals, including hard to get minerals like selenium, chromium, zinc.

5. B-12 Sublingual. A special note for seniors. The anemia of children is IRON deficiency. The anemia of seniors is B12 deficiency, also known as pernicious (meaning deadly) anemia.

The root cause of this in seniors is the attenuation of a protein carrier in the stomach as we age. That means that you could be taking plenty of B-12, but if you, in your senior years, don't have that "shuttle bus" protein to get it into your blood, it won't be absorbed.

To get B-12 into your blood quickly, seniors should take it in pill form *under the tongue.* When you put the B-12 sublingual tablet under your tongue, it will be immediately absorbed into your blood, totally bypassing your digestive system.

Supplements Which Relieve Stress:

The following are all non-prescription. You can use one or all at the same time. They are foods (eg. amino acids), vitamins, minerals, or herbs.

1. Calcium. The #1 mineral for relaxation of the body and muscles is calcium. Without sufficient calcium the muscles cannot relax.

2. GABA (an amino acid which helps relax the brain.)

3. Tryptophan or 5 HTP (an amino acid which triggers the "feel good" chemical, seratonin.)

4. Melatonin is the sleep hormone that is used for both stress relief and a good night's sleep. (A warm bath also stimulates melatonin production.)

5. DHEA also has anti-aging benefits.

6. Alpha Lipoic Acid helps reduce free radicals in the body

7. Magnesium is a mineral and is in a class of its own. It is called "Nature's Tranquilizer." It has over 300 different functions in the body. For the cancer survivor, it is used for relaxation.

8. Valerian is a natural herb that has been in use for hundreds of years for sleep.

I INTEND TO DO THE FOLLOWING:

---

10. How LOVE Heals

For the cancer survivor the toughest yet easiest path is 100% pure acceptance of not only your condition, but of life in general. Acceptance is the key. At first this may sound kind of strange and paradoxical, but the **non-resistance through acceptance and surrender is, in a way, love itself**.

There are many testimonials of cancer survivors who have taken this approach. It always works! One cancer survivor who did this said *"I feel truly ALIVE for the first time in my life!"* Another survivor recalls: *"From the depths of my suffering, I was suddenly flooded with gratitude!"*

I experienced this myself with a daily ritual. Here is a prayer I used every during my treatment and recovery process. Standing outdoors in a natural setting, I would glance around myself and say:

"This circle is my universe. Everything in this universe extends to the far extremes of what is; and my universe is perfect, is filled full of light, and is filled full of love."

There is a phenomenal psychological transition that occurs when you do this for a couple of months. You get the sense that **your thoughts** have the power to affect everything in your world. And, of course, they do!

So, if and when any negativity arises in your mind, and it probably will, just observe it, and then release it. Separate yourself from it. Realize that you never have to act on that negativity.

Remember: It's the very nature of the mind to conjure up these types of thoughts. This recognition and then release is all part of the acceptance and surrender process.

I INTEND TO USE THESE DAILY RITUALS AND AFFIRMATIONS:

APPENDIX

My Daily Menu

Mostly raw, these nutrient and fiber rich meals take 15-minutes or less to prepare. Enjoy!

For lunch and dinner, I keep the main entrée the same. What changes are the finger foods and condiments. This simple menu also keeps me regular and predictable.

Although I eat out several times a week, the following is my basic "at home" menu. Because it is NUTRIENT dense, it always satisfies. I don't have cravings for snack foods and sugars because I satisfy my daily nutritional needs this way.

Remember to *always eat protein first. Always drink liquids, 30-minutes before or after a meal.*

LUNCH

2-3 soft-boiled eggs, Season with salt, pepper and tumeric, stir, and drink like Chinese egg drop soup.

Green drink (see recipe on page 49).

1 TBSP Omega-3 Fish Oil (with DHA & EPA).

Lunch & Dinner Finger Foods

Enjoy slow dining with these favorite, nutrient and fiber rich foods. Eat foods of different colors!

Our daily table includes 5 small, pretty dishes. Each contains colorful, nutrient and fiber rich foods such as: plums, raisins, carob chips and chocolate (65% or more cocoa), dried cranberries, olives, and pickles. Enjoy as much as you like!

A serving tray holds a container of fresh ground almond (or peanut) butter, honey, jam, catsup, salsa and mustard. Note: nut butters are also protein. Enjoy 1-2 TBSP.

DINNER

½ - 1 tin of Sardines (from a clean, cold water source)

Serve on a bed of 2-3 TBSP cooked brown rice.

Green drink (see recipe on page 49).

1 TBSP Omega-3 Fish Oil (with DHA & EPA).

Remember to take your vitamins and supplements at meal time, unless otherwise directed.

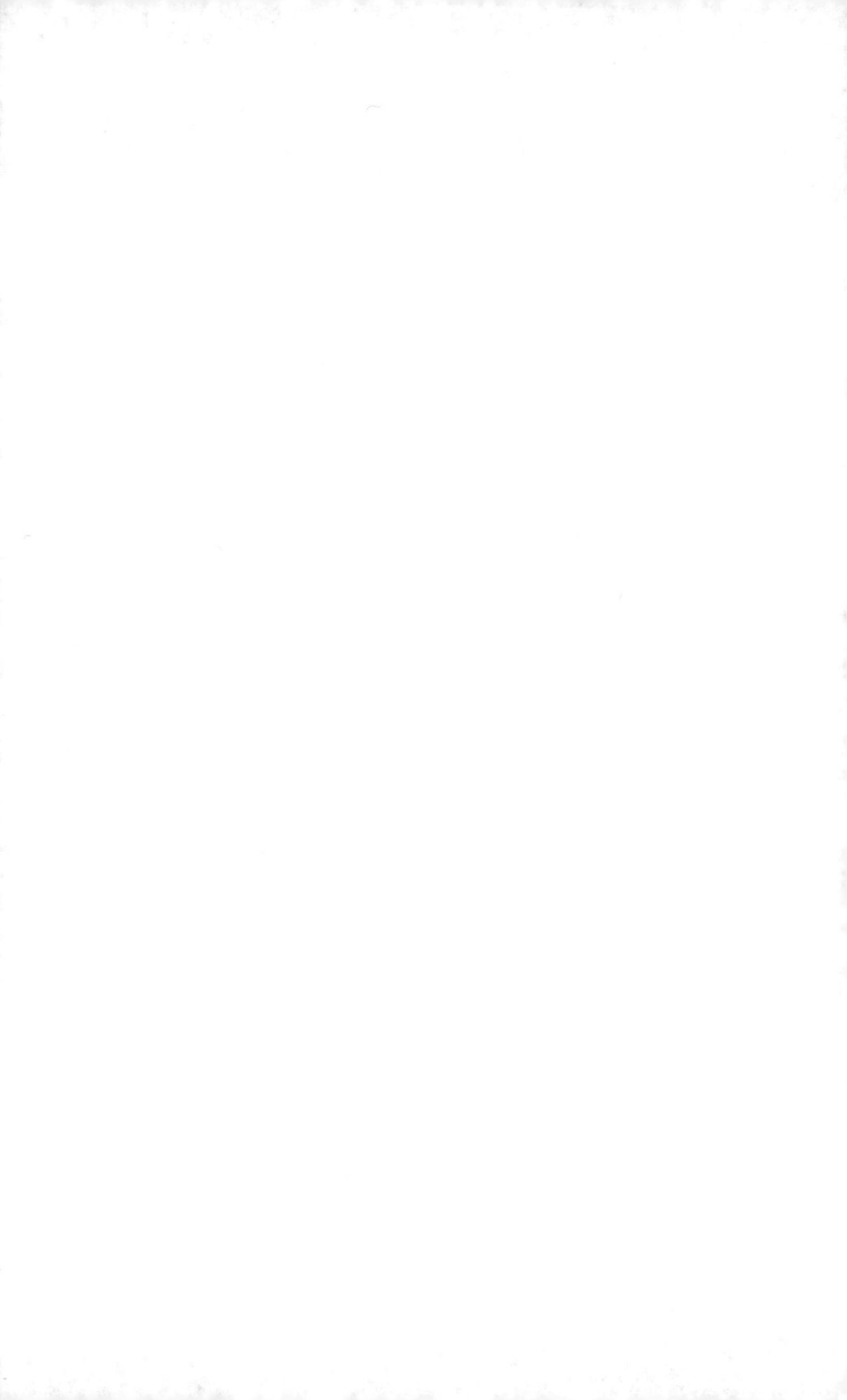

www.ingramcontent.com/pod-product-compliance
Lightning Source LLC
Chambersburg PA
CBHW060643290526
45793CB00001B/379